60 ESSENTIAL TIPS FOR LOSING WEIGHT

MICHAEL J. ROBERTS

TABLE OF CONTENTS

INTRODUCTION

There was then a time when the thought of losing weight did not exist in our society; people ate what their moms prepared for supper and went to work. The difference between that company and today's is that the work isn't done behind a computer screen but standing on the floor or in a dispersion center. Individuals work physically since that's the way to work; in reality, that's why we call it work! As a rule around this time, personalities can consume everything they require since they burn more calories than they use. Be that as it may, like all awesome things, this too has passed, and the development of today's world has liberated us from a circumstance:

Being bulky. Our way of life has altered, and our consolation has blown up ten times. As they say, each rose has its thorn, and in our society, the desire to live a comfortable life and work less has started to appear around the waistline. The awful thing about all of this is that you can simply frequently pick up more weight. It gets increasingly unsafe. Additional weight means illness. Whether it is diabetes or a heart infection, it'll show up if you do not do something. You wish to be proactive in picking up weight and making endeavors until you can't control it any longer. It is unlimited and instilled, but it contains a weight that does not hurt life. You'll be able to work out your back and stomach muscles. You should lose a little excess body fat right now. As society realizes what is happening—that we are, for the most part, bulky—individuals are striving to catch up and work remotely. They are trying to lose weight and live a more beneficial life. This eBook is your direct route to losing those 10 pounds we're all battling with. It's astonishing what little changes in your life can come from losing 10 pounds; it's all around eating right and being physically dynamic.

I

<u>DRINKING IS THE FIRST STEP</u>

<u>TOWARDS WEIGHT LOSS</u>

To begin with, individuals do not realize that what they drink is the primary step in losing 10 pounds. In truth, most individuals do not know that when they feel hungry, they may be dried out, and they are truly parched, not hungry. Water is surprising as well. Over 66% of your body weight is nothing but water. Usually, water plays an imperative part in weight control. So

Drink plenty of water. It is recommended that you just drink 8 glasses per day, but that will take you a while to work up to. Your body needs a lot of water. Water doesn't flush all the poisons out of your body, but it makes you feel better and more beneficial. After you drink a part of the water, you start to feel fit, and this is often the inspiration you would like to lose weight.

The best thing about water is that you'll be able to drink as much as you need since it has no calories at all. When you're drinking a parcel of water, you eat less as well since you won't feel hungry, although you're starving to death. Remember, if you feel hungry, attempt drinking a glass of water to begin with, and you'll realize you were likely fairly dried out and not hungry at all.

The entire 8 glasses a day rule is something you ought to endeavor for. perfect way">The most perfect way to do this and to degree your water admissions is to buy a jug from the sedate store or basic supply store that's outlined to hold exactly 8 glasses of water. These are great weight misfortune instruments since you'll fill them up and solidify them, and because they melt all through the day, you've got fresh and cold water. Or, on the off chance that you don't mind your water room temperature, you'll drink it that way as well. All that means is that you're getting the water your body needs.

TIP 2:

Commence the day by taking a fresh, clean glass of water. As before, as long as you wake at sunrise, gulp one down. This will help your body get going since it won't be combating dryness. Moreover, after you gulp a glass of water, you won't have to eat such an immense brunch. A glass of water wakes up all the belly-related juices in your body and gets it well-greased up. You'll be able to continuously have your morning coffee or tea, but be beyond any doubt about having a glass of water a short time later. Caffeine dehydrates you, and you need to ward off a lack of hydration.

TIP 3:

Take a glass of water occasionally when you sit down to eat. Water will normally make you feel more full, so you do not need to eat as much nourishment.

TIP 4:

Take a glass of water at the same time you eat as well. Take a sip after each nibble, and you'll feel full more rapidly, so you'll be able to take off from the table feeling fulfilled without feeling emotionally distended. Gulping water while you eat will also help your nourishment settle more rapidly, which, moreover, makes it easier for you to feel full quickly.

TIP 5:

Try your best to refrain from tonics. All tonics are sweetened with sugar. The more calories you reduce, the better. Plus, light pop is still pop. It may not contain much sugar, but It has chemicals and other ingredients that are unacceptable for your body. If you drink tonics, test them with a glass of water. Recall that brew also dehydrates you. Caffeine-free tonics still contain small amounts of caffeine as well as sugar, so they aren't much more beneficial.

TIP 6:

Fruit punches are also not as healthy as people think. Fruit punches also accommodate a lot of sugar. If you crave a glass of extract, drink fresh extract instead of juice with artificial flavors and colors. It would be better if you could produce your raw juice. Just make sure you don't add too much dextrose, which will add calories. Instead of taking juice, drink more fruit. Fruits provide your body with the necessary amount of fiber and vitamins.

TIP 7:

Feel free to drink tea and coffee. They are practically harmless if you do not add a lot of cream and sugar to them. It is cream and sugar that cause you to gain weight. Think of it this way: When you drink a cup of coffee or tea with cream and two sugar cubes, you're essentially eating one piece of chocolate cake at a time. Now think about how many pieces of cake you eat while drinking a Venti Starbucks Latte.

TIP 8:

If you must drink tea and coffee, try siping them black. Black tea or coffee is healthy, as long as you neutralize the caffeine in your body with a large glass of water. Caffeine is also bad for you because it affects body functions, such as metabolism.

Another type of tea that you can drink freely is green tea. Green tea has been used medicinally in China for over 4,000 years. It helps the digestive system and can help relieve an overfull stomach. It is linked to a reduced risk of cancer.

TIP 9:

If you can say no to alcohol, even better. Alcoholic drinks are not good for your health. Although a glass of red wine has some heart-healthy benefits, it mostly just makes you gain weight. Beer is especially fattening. Cocktails are fattening, depending on their ingredients. For example: whiskey and Coke. Whiskey may not be fattening, but Coke certainly is. Additionally, after a few glasses of wine, most people experience cravings, and when you feel a little drunk and hungry, you won't be able to make rational decisions about your diet, and that's often the case. late at night, right before you pass out overnight—drinking alcohol, eating too much. The overall combination is not good.

TIP 10:

In the event that you must drink wine, attempt brut. Brut is superior to dessert wine since pudding wine accommodates a bunch of sugar! Brut wines contain a little sugar, but most of it has matured into liquor, and in terms of weight pick-up, bruts are superior.

TIP 11:

Another word on coffee—that's not essentially terrible but more curious than anything. A few individuals have detailed that when they drank dark coffee sometime recently while working out, they lost more weight. There's no logical confirmation to back this, but nutritionists accept it may be caused by the body being constrained to depend on fat for fuel. Hello, it's worth trying if you'll be able to stand dark coffee. Keep in mind to drink a bounty of water during your workout!

TIP 12:

Sustain a crucial distance from drinking over-the-top portions of coffee because it desensitizes your body to the normal fat-burning impacts that caffeine has. One or two mugs (if the day's truly moderate to start) max.

III

HEALTHY EATING AND WEIGHT LOSS

Affirm that when most individuals think about losing weight and eating, they think about counting calories. Well, tragically, all of the prevailing fashion diets out there tend to cause individuals to gain weight. Why? Since they starve them to death, the individual inevitably breaks down and eats everything in sight since they are so darn hungry. They also deny them the nourishment that they cherish. This is often not a way to lose weight, nor is it a way to live. You merely cause yourself to push, which causes you to gain weight!

So, in eating, there are a couple of tips that you can just take after each day, and they're not going to deny you the nourishments that you just cherish, but treat those nourishments as extravagance things so you appreciate them that much more.

TIP 13:

Eat new natural products and greens that contain a lofty moisture. These are nutriments like a tomato plants, melons, muskmelons, chinese-gooseberry, and grapes—you get the concept. All of those new and tasty, succulent natural products and greens are great for you. These things contain around 90 to 95% water, so you'll be able to eat a part of them, and they will fill you up without including the pounds.

TIP 14:

Eat new raw produce rather than treated natural produce. Anything that's primed has more sugar. Primed and canned natural products, moreover, don't have as much fiber as new natural products.

TIP 15:

Raise your bulk consumption as much as viable. This commonly entails taking more fruits and veggies.

TIP 16:

Greens are your buddies when it comes to dropping pounds. There are tons of choices here, and you will indeed need to undertake a few you haven't had in the past. The verdant green assortments are the finest, and you continuously need to work in a serving of mixed greens once you can. Servings of mixed greens are pressed with supplements, as long as you do not pour as much dressing on them and stack them with as much cheese. The verdant greens also have a parcel of characteristic water.

TIP 17:

Be astute about what you eat. Do not eat what you want to eat. Creatures eat intuitively; individuals eat when they know their body truly needs it. Do not be a drive-thru.

TIP 18:

Observe everything you expend, from the nourishment itself to what you beat it with.

Garnishments and flavorings can disrupt a sound dinner since they are ordinarily high in fat.

TIP 19:

Get a handle on the sweet tooth. This isn't cruel; you can't have your desserts; do not eat them as a feast. Continuously keep in mind that these desserts end up in a range that you simply do not need them to include. Do not deny yourself either, even though, at that point, you'll eat twice as many as you ought to.

TIP 20:

Set dinner hours and adhere to them. Attempt to have your suppers at particular hours and eat them at those hours. A feeding design will assist you in controlling what you eat and after you eat it.

Moreover, it truly is better to have five little suppers

a day instead of one or two gigantic suppers. Fair

feeding once a day makes your body feel just as if it

is starved, which packs on fat rather than utilizing it

as fuel. Also, do not hold up until you are starving to

eat. This, as it were, makes you indulge until you're

stuffed.

Eat as if you were hungry. Be beyond any doubt to drink a glass of water, to begin with, to decide on the off chance that you are hungry or on the off chance that you're truly parched. Numerous individuals have the propensity to eat when they see nourishment. It isn't cruel; they are hungry; they just need to eat it. Do not eat anything you're offered unless you truly are hungry. If you are feeling you must eat it out of being a neighborly, fair snack, do not have a supper.

TIP 22:

Try not to snack between dinners, but if you must have a snack, make sure it's solid. If you are in transit, try to explore solid snacks and not canned food.

TIP 23:

Veggies make incredible snacks. They can get you through the starvation throbs on the off chance that you're having them. Carrots are extraordinary since they fulfill starvation and are stuffed with supplements.

TIP 24:

Checking kilocalories can be a great thought for persons who want to nourish themselves. On the off chance that it could be bundled nourishment, it'll contain the sum of calories recorded on the bundling. Be beyond any doubt about paying consideration to parcel sizes in terms of calories. One Otis Spunkmeyer biscuit is for two servings, so you ought to double the calories recorded. Maybe usually when nourishment makers feel unreliable and you cannot drop into their trap.

TIP 25:

Sweat out the added kilocalories by the conclusion of the week. If you are feeling you've splurged as well this week, be beyond any doubt to go to the exercise center or go strolling a little longer to work off those additional calories you have expended.

TIP 26:

Remain absent from all things browned. On the off chance that it is breaded, it is superior that it be prepared. Fricasseed nourishments are submerged in fat and oil. Indeed, after the abundance of oil has been depleted, there's still oil retained in the nourishment thing itself.

TIP 27:

Don't leave out food. You must eat a minimum of a complete meal a day, but five small dinners are ideal. This will prevent you from feeling starved all day, leading to starvation.

TIP 28:

Rather similar to natural produce, new greens are superior to those that are canned. It is indeed superior on the off chance that you'll be able to eat your veggies raw. After you cook them, you cook them without the supplements. If you must cook them, attempt to bubble them to the point that there's still a little freshness to them. Moreover, do not douse them in butter. If you'll purchase natural and pesticide-free veggies, that's indeed superior.

TIP 29:

Don't eat up more than one egg per day. It is best on the off chance that you'll limit your egg admissions to three a week.

TIP 30:

Chocolate ought to be treated as an extravagance. Purchase the great stuff and, as it were, eat them each once in a short time. If you truly savor each piece, you'll have that much more delight in eating them, and they will indeed taste way better.

TIP 31:

Eat diets from all diet groups daily. This is a great way to ensure you get all the minerals your body wants and prevent any nutritive deficiencies. Also, don't always eat similar meals. Experiment so you don't get bored with the same old diet.

TIP 32:

Try to eat breakfast within an hour of waking up. It's the best way to give your body the boost it needs. Don't wait until you're really hungry. Breakfast is important, but you don't need to eat too much. The idea is that you fast by not stopping all night long.

TIP 33:

Your meal has to include all food groups, including carbs. Your meal should weigh around 50 to 55 pounds. Sugars are an excellent source of vitality. These diets that ban carbs are harming you and only making you crave more. Your diet will leave you lacking in just about anything.

TIP 34:

Protein has to only make up 25–30% of your meal. There is also much emphasis on meat as the major part of your meal. It should be regarded as a side dish rather than a main dish.

TIP 35:

Fat must constitute 15-20% of your meals. That's all the fat your body needs. Much of this will appear in your diet in the form of cream, sugar, etc.

TIP 36:

Eat more wing meat than ruddy meat. Wing meat incorporates chicken, angle, and a few other sorts of poultry. Ruddy meat incorporates hamburgers and pork.

TIP 37:

Attempt to go as veggie-loving as you'll be able. This truly could be a more beneficial way of life, even if you can't cut meat out totally. The more natural products and veggies you'll be able to eat, The more meat you cut out, the more fat you'll be able to gain. cut out of your slime as well. In any case, protein is imperative, so be certain that your alternative permits you to preserve great protein levels.

TIP 38:

Hamburger bread is sweetened, but high-fiber brown bread is far superior. These hamburgers are another way to add more grain to your kilocalories, and they also have great protein content.

TIP 39:

Pork does not help with weight misfortune in any way. The less pork you eat, the better off you may be when attempting to lose weight. Pork incorporates a tall fat substance and contains nutrients such as bacon, ham, and frankfurter.

TIP 40:

Constrain your sugar intake as much as is conceivable. If you must have a sweetener in your coffee or tea, attempt to discover a counterfeit sweetener that you just do not know the taste of. Be that as it may, these things are not all that sound either and ought to be constrained as well.

TIP 41:

Attempt brushing five to six times a day. These are those little dinners we examined prior. A few individuals lose weight way better when they never feel hungry, and brushing on sound nourishment can do this for them. Also, it keeps your digestion system working, which is able to burn fat normally.

TIP 42:

Do not stress about cheating, but do not deceive for supper. Eat desserts and your favorite deceived nourishment for the flavor as it were. If you need dessert after supper, share one with the whole family. You'll get the flavor, but not the pounds.

TIP 43:

Observe your cellulite entry. Each cellulite gram has 9 calories. If you know your add-up to calories at that point, you'll be able to work out the sum of fat in those things.

TIP 44:

Lessen your saline ingestion, and try cutting back the quantity of saline you use in half. Salt is one of the principal sources of obesity.

III

CHANGE YOUR COOKING HABITS

TO LOSE WEIGHT

Here are a few hints to aid you drop those first 10 pounds just by changing the way you prepare food. The way foods are cooked also has a lot to do with whether they are healthy or not.

TIP 45:

In preference to broiling them in oil, attempt flame broiling them. Barbecuing doesn't require all the fats and oils required for singing, and your nourishment isn't exposed to these substances while cooking.

TIP 46:

Utilize a slippy broiling skillet shower so you do not use oil. Likewise, slippery plates do not require as much if there is any oil.

TIP 47:

Bubble greens in place of simmering them. You'll also steam them because that's likely the most advantageous way to keep supplements like lettuce, cole floret, broccoli, and carrots.

TIP 48:

Be cautious of no-fat and low-fat nourishment things. There are numerous of these nourishment things on the showcase, but they are not precisely sound. Numerous of these nourishment foods utilize a few sorts of chemicals or carbohydrates to sweeten them so that they taste superior. Be that as it may, the body turns these chemicals and carbohydrates into sugar within the body, which implies they are still getting turned into fat.

TIP 49:

Do not drop casualties on crash diets. These are awful for you and do more harm than good in the long run. The short-term results are that you will regularly simply lose a couple of pounds, but once you give them up at that point, everything comes back, and your weight is more awful at the moment. You cannot survive on a crash-slim down, and you inevitably

TIP 50:

Chew your nourishment at least 8 to 12 times, whether it is fluid nourishment, desserts, or ice cream. This includes spitting at the nourishment that digests the sugar. When nourishment isn't eaten appropriately and is gulped, you fill your stomach with nourishment that isn't prepared to be processed, and at that point, you do not surrender the well-being benefits it merely requires.

TIP 51:

Once you are simmering with oil, use great additional refined olive oil. It is more costly than cooking oil, but the well-being benefits are much superior, and it is worth the toll. Olive oil has been correlated with a reduced chance of coronary heart infection and makes a difference by extending the

flexibility of the blood vessel dividers, which

diminishes the chance of heart assault and stroke.

IV

<u>WORKING OUT TO LOSE WEIGHT</u>

There are two things that you simply must do to lose weight, and one of those is to eat right and fill your body with great, clean water. The other thing you have to do is get your body moving. You don't need to buy an exercise center membership to induce exercise. There are a few things you'll be able to do daily that will offer assistance to kick-start your body into losing weight, and there are a few workouts you'll be able to do on your claim to lose weight.

TIP 52:

After you start working out, whether at home or in an exercise center, do not be debilitated on the off chance that you do not see it coming about right away. It takes more than a week to get your body into shape and to start making progress. Several individuals make the mistake of accepting that their workout isn't working when it only takes a small bit of time.

If you thrust your body as well once you get started exercising, you'll end up with wounds. Your bones, joints, and tendons are not arranged for the effort you're putting into them. Do not think that on the off chance that you truly thrust yourself so hard for several workouts, you'll lose cash; shockingly, the body doesn't work this way. Moderate and unfaltering win the race when it comes to working out.

TIP 53:

Check your weight after you begin working out, but do not use it as a guide to how much body weight you're losing. Your body weight changes all through the day. If you check your weight each day, you will, as it were, end up getting debilitated.

TIP 54:

perfect way">The most perfect way to know in case you're losing weight is by the fit of your dress. If you begin to feel as though, even though you're coasting in your dress at that point, you know you're eating and working out, which is doing you a few great things. Another way to know on the off chance that you're losing weight is in case you'll start moving, where you buckle your belt more often than not; of course, more tightly is superior.

TIP 55:

Once you occasionally examine your body weight and the fit of your dress, remunerate yourself. Purchase yourself a few modern running shoes or an unused pair of pants. This will offer assistance to keep you propelled as you seek after your weight-misfortune objectives.

TIP 56:

Select a workout schedule that suits your way of life. Everyone encompasses a diverse way of life and a different profession. There's no set time that you just ought to or ought not to work out. If you like to work out late, you go to bed since it is unwinding for you at that point. If you like to work early in the morning since it makes a difference that you wake up at that point, that's extraordinary too. Some individuals like to work on their lunch break to take a break from the stretch of their work or since that's the only time they have available.

TIP 57:

Collect data on workouts and simple things you'll be able to do from home. There are tons of broad inquiries about accessible workouts, and you'll be able to select what will help you the most to meet your weight reduction goals. Browse the Web or pick up a few books on wellbeing and work out from your local bookstore or library to memorize more and how to burn off the required number of calories you're attempting to burn each week.

TIP 58:

Attempt to discover a workout buddy. This ought to be somebody who is as committed to working out and losing weight as you are. One of the points of interest in finding a committed partner is that you just have somebody to keep you mindful of them. The information that someone is holding up on you makes it simpler for you to get out of bed and go work out with them. You wouldn't need to stand up for your workout buddy, would you?

TIP 59:

Three days of 30 miniature grills will assist you in preserving your weight, but you wish at the very least 4 days of 30 miniature workouts to start to lose weight, and 5 days a week is indeed way

better.

TIP 60:

Supposing that you have a job where you sit the

whole time, stand up, and stretch each half hour or

so, the majority of today's jobs require you to sit in

front of a computer. In case you've got a job like

this, make it a point to move each one so regularly.